MUSCULAR DEGENERATION DIET COOKBOOK:

FOR NEWLY DIAGNOSED

Complete Beginner Procedures On Food Recipes, Guided Meal Plans, And Healthy Lifestyle Tips To Manage, Strive, And Live Well With AMD

DR. EMMY BROOKS

ABOUT THIS BOOK

This comprehensive guide aims to simplify the Muscular Degeneration Diet, providing practical recipes, clear procedures, and valuable insights to make the journey accessible for novices. From understanding the condition to creating lifelong habits, this cookbook serves as a supportive resource for managing muscular degeneration through a well-guided dietary approach.

In the realm of health and well-being, the "Muscular Degeneration Diet Cookbook" stands as a beacon of knowledge, offering a comprehensive guide to understanding and managing the intricate relationship between diet and muscular degeneration. The introduction sets the stage by emphasizing the crucial role nutrition plays in this condition, inviting readers into a journey of discovery that extends far beyond traditional dietary guidelines.

Delving into the heart of the matter, the book elucidates the basics of a muscular degeneration diet, unraveling the nutritional requirements essential for maintaining eye health. It masterfully highlights the significance of key nutrients and their role in combating the effects of this condition, elevating the discourse to a level where readers gain a profound understanding of the symbiotic connection between food and eye wellness.

As the narrative progresses, the focus shifts to building a foundation with essential ingredients, emphasizing the incorporation of antioxidant-rich foods and the importance of omega-3 fatty acids. This section serves as a practical guide, equipping readers with tangible tools to enhance their diet and fortify their bodies against the challenges posed by muscular degeneration.

The culinary journey continues with meal planning strategies, offering insights into creating balanced and nutrient-dense meals. The book not only provides theoretical knowledge but also practical tips for weekly meal planning, empowering readers to take charge of their dietary choices with confidence and intention.

Turning the page, the spotlight intensifies on cooking techniques that maximize nutrition retention. It skillfully navigates the complexities of optimal cooking methods, ensuring that readers can derive the maximum benefits from their culinary endeavors. This section goes beyond mere recipes, fostering a deeper understanding of the science behind cooking for eye health.

Superfoods take center stage in the subsequent chapters, bringing a burst of vitality to the dietary landscape. The book meticulously explores foods beneficial for muscular degeneration, offering practical ways to incorporate these superfoods into daily meals. The emphasis on variety and accessibility underscores the book's commitment to making healthy eating both enjoyable and feasible.

The culinary adventure unfolds with dedicated chapters on breakfast, lunch, and dinner, presenting quick, nutrient-packed recipes that cater to different tastes and lifestyles. From wholesome one-pot dinners to eye-nourishing breakfast smoothies, each section is a testament to the book's mission: to provide readers with a diverse repertoire of recipes that align with a muscular degeneration diet.

Addressing the nuances of dining out and social situations, the book becomes a companion in navigating restaurant menus and making informed choices at gatherings. It empowers readers to enjoy social occasions without compromising their commitment to eye health, fostering a sense of confidence in their ability to maintain a balanced diet in various settings.

The inclusion of a chapter on nutritional supplements underscores the book's holistic approach. It demystifies supplement options, urging readers to engage in informed discussions with healthcare professionals to tailor their supplementation to individual needs.

As the journey nears its end, the book underscores the importance of a long-term commitment to eye health. It celebrates successes and guides overcoming challenges, cementing its status as an indispensable resource for those on the path to sustained well-being.

In essence, the "Muscular Degeneration Diet Cookbook" transcends its title, emerging as an engaging and elevating narrative that empowers readers to embrace a lifestyle that seamlessly integrates culinary delights with the pursuit of eye health.

DISCLAIMER

This book's content is solely intended for general informative purposes. About the availability, applicability, correctness, completeness, and trustworthiness of the data or recipes in this book, the author provides no guarantees of any sort, either stated or implied. You bear full responsibility for any reliance you may have on such material.

The advice, diagnosis, or treatment provided by a qualified medical expert is not to be replaced by this cookbook. When in doubt about a medical problem, never hesitate to consult your doctor or another trained healthcare professional. Never ignore medical advice from professionals or put off getting it because of something you've read in this book.

At the time of publishing, the author of this book has taken reasonable steps to guarantee that the information is correct and current. He does not, however, guarantee that the data will be error-free or that it will satisfy any certain performance or quality standards. Any negative repercussions that may arise from using or applying the material in this book are not the responsibility of the author, publisher, or distributor.

In this book, references or mentions of individuals, products, websites, organizations, or other names are for informational purposes only and do not imply endorsement or affiliation with the author. The author has no control over the nature, content, and availability of referenced or mentioned entities. Any reliance on such information is at the reader's own risk.

The inclusion of any references does not necessarily imply a recommendation or endorse the views expressed within them. The author or publisher shall not be liable for any loss or damage arising out of or in connection with, the use of this book.

INTRODUCTION

Understanding Muscular Degeneration:

Age-related macular degeneration (AMD), also known as muscular degeneration, is a degenerative eye disease that mostly affects the macula, or center portion of the retina. Loss of central vision due to this degenerative process might impair one's ability to notice tiny details, recognize people, and carry out daily chores. It's important to investigate the fundamental causes of muscle degeneration to fully understand its subtleties.

The aging process is one of the main factors contributing to muscle degeneration because it causes the cells and tissues in the macula to break down. Important roles are also played by genetics, lifestyle decisions, and environmental variables in the development and course of this illness. Dry AMD, which is defined by the slow degeneration of macular cells, and wet AMD, which is characterized by the formation of aberrant blood vessels beneath the macula, are the two primary forms of muscle degeneration.

Recognizing the symptoms of muscle degeneration, such as distorted or blurred vision, trouble reading, and difficulties identifying faces, is essential to comprehend the complexities of the condition. For the early diagnosis and treatment of muscle degeneration, routine eye exams are crucial. Equipped with this understanding, people can take proactive measures to deal with the illness, concentrating especially on dietary changes that support a comprehensive management strategy.

A Synopsis of Muscle Degeneration

A thorough understanding of muscle degeneration entails investigating the many phases of the illness, methods of diagnosis, and possible therapies. Three phases are commonly used to describe the evolution of muscle degeneration: early AMD, moderate AMD, and advanced AMD.

Early stages may show very few symptoms, therefore it's important for those who are at risk to get regular eye exams.

OCT and fluorescein angiography are two diagnostic techniques that offer fine-grained pictures of the retina and blood vessels. Knowing how to use these diagnostic techniques can help people and medical professionals monitor the development of muscle degeneration and choose the best course of action.

Depending on the kind and level of muscle degeneration, many treatment approaches are available. Although there isn't a cure at this time, management techniques include changing one's lifestyle, using prescription drugs, and occasionally having surgery. By providing people with the knowledge they need to make educated decisions regarding their eye health, this thorough summary opens the door to a proactive strategy for treating muscle degeneration.

Diet is Important for Managing the Condition:

For those looking to take charge of their eye health, it is critical to understand the critical role that nutrition plays in controlling muscle degeneration. It has been demonstrated that a diet high in nutrients and well-balanced can significantly decrease the course of AMD and improve general eye health. Customizing a diet to meet the specific requirements of people with muscle degeneration requires an understanding of the particular nutrients that sustain ocular function.

Antioxidants, including zinc, lutein, and vitamins C and E, are crucial for preserving eye health and reducing oxidative stress, which is a major contributor to the onset of muscle degeneration. Flaxseed and salmon, which are high in omega-3 fatty acids, also aid in maintaining retinal function.

A diet high in fish, nuts, whole grains, dark leafy greens, and colorful fruits and vegetables serves as the cornerstone of a nutritional plan to address muscle atrophy.

An ideal diet for people with this eye ailment also takes into account portion control, moderation in the consumption of saturated fats and cholesterol, and staying hydrated.

Knowing the underlying causes, phases, and current treatments of muscle degeneration is essential to understanding the condition. A thorough summary helps people to make decisions regarding the health of their eyes. It is impossible to overestimate the significance that nutrition plays in managing muscle degeneration because a diet rich in nutrients and well-balanced is essential for maintaining eye health and delaying the advancement of the problem. Equipped with this understanding, people can set out on a personalized, guided dietary path for the best possible eye health and general well-being.

CHAPTER ONE

AN INTRODUCTION TO A DIET FOR MUSCULAR DEGENERATION

The Dietary Needs for the Degeneration of Muscle

Keeping up a diet designed to combat muscle deterioration requires choosing specific nutrients carefully because they are essential for maintaining eye health. Taking a comprehensive approach is necessary to guarantee that the body gets a variety of key vitamins and minerals. One of the main things to think about for those who are suffering from muscle deterioration is adding antioxidants, omega-3 fatty acids, and certain vitamins such as A, C, and E.

Fruits and vegetables are rich in antioxidants, which are essential for preventing oxidative stress, which is a major cause of muscle deterioration. To guarantee a varied dose of antioxidants, include berries, spinach, and carrots, among other colorful foods.

These potent substances aid in the neutralization of free radicals, protecting the sensitive ocular cells from harm.

Omega-3 fatty acids are important for maintaining eye health. They are particularly present in fatty fish like salmon and trout. These good fats support overall stability and function by supporting the structural integrity of the cell membranes of the eyes. Omega-3s can be obtained from plants in the form of flaxseeds and chia seeds, which are good options for people who may not like fish.

Essential allies in the fight against muscle degeneration are vitamins A, C, and E. Sweet potatoes and kale are two examples of foods high in vitamin A that help to keep the retina healthy. Vitamin C-rich foods like bell peppers and citrus fruits strengthen the immune system and promote the synthesis of collagen, which is essential for maintaining eye structure. By lowering oxidative stress, vitamin E—which is abundant in nuts and seeds—supports the general health of the eyes.

Achieving equilibrium among these many nutrients is crucial. Even though each has a specific function, together they strengthen the body's resistance against muscle deterioration. Developing a diet plan that consists of a range of foods high in nutrients guarantees that the body gets a wide range of nutrients that are essential for eye health.

Essential Elements for Eye Health

Before delving into the particulars of essential nutrients for eye health, it is critical to comprehend how each one supports the preservation of ideal eyesight and the prevention of muscle deterioration. Carotenoids called lutein and zeaxanthin, which are present in leafy greens like kale and spinach, are crucial for shielding the eyes from potentially damaging high-energy light rays.

Zinc is another essential vitamin that can be found in large amounts in meat, dairy products, and legumes.

Zinc is essential for the movement of vitamin A from the liver to the retina, which helps the eyes adapt to low light. Consuming meals high in zinc guarantees a consistent intake of this essential element.

Furthermore, it is critical to maintain a sufficient diet of vitamins C and E. These vitamins function as potent antioxidants and are found in fruits, vegetables, nuts, and seeds. Specifically, vitamin C supports the body's general defense against oxidative stress by helping to regenerate other antioxidants.

One can approach the process of including these essential nutrients in everyday meals methodically. For example, consuming a nutrient-dense smoothie made with spinach, berries, and almonds first thing in the morning offers a concentrated amount of lutein, zeaxanthin, and vitamin E. Lunchtime can be centered around a vibrant salad with vegetables high in vitamins A and C, and dinner could be a portion of fatty fish or plant-based omega-3 fatty acid substitutes.

People can easily incorporate these components into their diets by decomposing nutrient requirements into doable meal options. This method not only makes the procedure easier for beginners, but it also guarantees a regular and uniform intake of the necessary ingredients required to keep the eyes healthy and fight muscle deterioration.

CHAPTER TWO

LAYING THE GROUNDWORK: CRUCIAL ELEMENTS

Including Foods Rich in Antioxidants:

A Muscular Degeneration Diet Cookbook's core is the deliberate inclusion of foods high in antioxidants. Antioxidants are essential in the fight against oxidative stress, which is a major contributor to the deterioration of muscles. Beginners should concentrate on including a range of vibrant fruits and vegetables in their daily meals because these selections frequently have high antioxidant content. Berries rich in antioxidants like anthocyanins and vitamin C, such as blueberries, strawberries, and raspberries, are great options.

Furthermore, leafy greens like kale and spinach are superfoods because they include a wide range of antioxidants including lutein and zeaxanthin.

These substances are essential for people with muscle degeneration because they have been particularly associated with maintaining eye health. A useful strategy for beginners would be to use these items to make colorful salads or smoothies for a tasty and eye-catching antioxidant boost.

Additionally, adding nuts and seeds to meals—like walnuts, chia seeds, and almonds—can improve their antioxidant profile. Vitamin E, another strong antioxidant that supports general eye health, is available from these sources. Adding these nuts and seeds to salads, yogurt, or high-energy snacks is a simple way for beginners to include them in their diet.

To summarize, to have a well-rounded experience with the Muscular Degeneration Diet Cookbook, beginners should focus on a colorful, wide array of foods that are rich in antioxidants and include them in different meals and snacks.

Acids Omega-3 and Their Function:

Omega-3 fatty acids are an integral part of a Muscular Degeneration Diet Cookbook and are vital for sustaining eye health. Novices need to know that certain fatty acids, especially docosahexaenoic acid (DHA) and eicosapentaenoic acid (EPA), have neuroprotective and anti-inflammatory properties that slow down the deterioration of muscles.

Focusing on adding fatty fish, such as salmon, mackerel, and sardines, to your diet is a sensible first step for beginners. These fish are excellent providers of DHA and EPA.

One easy and delicious approach to incorporating omega-3 fatty acids into daily meals is to bake or grill fish fillets. If fish is not to everyone's taste, omega-3 supplements made from algae or fish oil can be used as a substitute to make sure that these important fats are consumed in sufficient amounts.

For beginners, plant-based sources of omega-3 fatty acids like walnuts, chia seeds, and flaxseeds are also great choices. These are a great way to increase omega-3 levels without being meat-based or dairy-based. They may be added to cereals, smoothies, or salads.

Finally, to ensure a well-rounded and pleasurable approach to maintaining eye health, beginners should give special attention to adding omega-3 fatty acids to their Muscular Degeneration Diet Cookbook from both fish and plant-based sources.

CHAPTER THREE

ORGANIZING MEALS TO PREVENT MUSCULAR DEGENERATION

Making Nutrient-Dense, Balanced Meals:

Recognizing Nutritional Needs:

Meals high in nutrients that promote overall eye health become essential for managing muscle degeneration. Antioxidants such as vitamins A, C, and E, along with minerals like zinc, are important nutrients. These nutrients are essential for preserving eye health and reducing the rate at which muscle degeneration progresses.

Adding Vibrant Fruits and Vegetables:

Keeping your attention on a rainbow of fruits and veggies is an easy and successful strategy. Color variations correspond to different nutritional profiles. For instance, lutein and zeaxanthin, which are known to have eye-protective qualities, are abundant in leafy greens like spinach and kale. Vibrant carrots, bell peppers, and berries can increase the diversity of nutrients in your meals.

Lean Proteins to Support Your Muscles:

Proteins are necessary to keep muscles healthy. Choose lean protein sources including fish, lentils, and legumes, as well as skinless chicken. These offer a healthy ratio of amino acids without having too much-saturated fat. Consuming omega-3 fatty acids from foods like flaxseeds or fatty fish can help improve the general health of your muscles and eyes.

Whole Grains Provide Long-Term Energy:

Including whole grains in your diet guarantees a consistent release of energy and supplies vital nutrients such as fiber, magnesium, and B vitamins. For general well-being, choose foods like quinoa, brown rice, and oats. These grains help people with muscle degeneration maintain an active lifestyle by helping to stabilize blood sugar levels and helping to minimize fatigue.

Good Fats for Uptake of Nutrients:

Healthy fats should not be avoided because they aid in the absorption of nutrients. Omega-3 fatty acids and monounsaturated fats can be found in abundance in avocados, nuts, seeds, and olive oil. In addition to being good for eye health, these fats aid in the absorption of fat-soluble vitamins including A, D, and E.

Drinking Water and Herbal Teas:

It is common to undervalue the importance of maintaining proper hydration, even for eye health. Encourage hydration all day long. Herbal drinks, especially those high in antioxidants such as green tea, can be a delicious and refreshing addition that improves the general health of people suffering from muscle degeneration.

Mealtime Routine and Portion Control:

It's important to keep portion sizes in check to avoid overindulging and to advance general wellness. To ensure that the body receives a consistent supply of nutrients without taxing the digestive system, aim for smaller, more frequent meals throughout the day. This method promotes energy levels and helps to normalize blood sugar levels.

Weekly Meal Planning Techniques:

Preparation and Purchasing Groceries:

Make a menu in advance of your weekly meal planning by allocating time for it. Take into account your dietary preferences and goals, making sure to include a range of foods to guarantee a well-rounded diet. Make a shopping list as soon as your menu is ready to help you save time when you visit the grocery store. Making a plan guarantees that you have all the components on hand and lowers the likelihood of impulsive purchases.

Using Batch Cooking to Save Time:

Make your week easier by implementing batch cooking into your daily schedule. Prepare staple foods like grains, proteins, and vegetables in greater amounts and store them in portion-controlled containers.

This helps to create balanced meals throughout the week by saving time and offering the convenience of having pre-prepared items on hand.

Diverse and Adaptable: Accept diversity in your diet to avoid boredom and guarantee a wide range of nutrients. To make your meals interesting, switch up the grains, veggies, and kinds of protein you eat. Furthermore, be adaptable with your plan. Having backup plans or quick, wholesome go-to meals on hand might help you maintain your focus even on the busiest of days.

Mindful Food Practices: To improve digestion and the dining experience overall, adopt mindful eating practices. Eat mindfully, chew slowly, and pay attention to your body's signals of hunger and fullness with each bite. This method aids in preventing overeating in addition to improving digestion.

Observing and Modifying: Evaluate your body's reaction to the eating plan regularly. Keep an eye on your digestion, energy levels, and any changes in your general health. If necessary, seek advice from a nutritionist or healthcare provider to modify your strategy in light of your unique requirements and any particular factors associated with muscular degeneration.

Putting Together a Support Network:

Include friends, family, and support networks in your meal-planning process. In addition to making the experience more fun, interacting with others fosters an environment that is conducive to establishing and sustaining healthy eating practices. Promote candid discussion about preferences and difficulties so that you may work together to overcome any barriers to following the meal plan.

Examining and Honoring Advancement:

Take some time to consider your path and acknowledge your advancements. Acknowledge the improvements in your eating patterns and general health. Recognizing modest successes boosts motivation and emphasizes the need to stick to a healthy diet designed to assist those with muscle degeneration.

CHAPTER FOUR

COOKING METHODS FOR OPTIMAL NUTRITION

Ideal Cooking Techniques:

When it comes to preparing meals for people on a Muscular Degeneration diet, cooking is essential. Proper cooking techniques not only improve the taste of the food but also aid in the preservation of vital nutrients, guaranteeing a balanced and nutritious meal. It's critical for beginners starting this culinary adventure to comprehend and use cooking methods that optimize nutrition without sacrificing flavor.

The usage of steaming as a favored cooking method is one of the essential factors to take into account. Vegetables can be cooked gently and effectively while maintaining their colorful hues and nutrient content by steaming. By purchasing a basic, reasonably priced steamer basket, beginners can effortlessly integrate steaming into their daily regimen.

This simple gadget may be set over a pot of boiling water to cook veggies while the steam preserves their essential elements. Vegetables high in antioxidants and vitamins essential for eye health, such as broccoli, spinach, and kale, benefit greatly from steaming.

Sautéing using healthful oils is another crucial method that new cooks should use. When using standard cooking oils that are heavy in saturated fats, choose heart-healthy substitutes like avocado or olive oil. These oils offer a delicious depth of flavor in addition to being a vital source of monounsaturated fats that support general health. Beginners can begin by preheating a small skillet with oil, adding their favorite vegetables, and sautéing them gently until they are the required tenderness. This technique adds a wonderful flavor to the food while preserving nutrients.

Another simple method that even beginners can use to enhance the nutritional value of their meals is grilling. Food that has been grilled acquires a distinct smoky flavor without the need for excessive oils or fats. It works especially well on lean protein sources like skinless chicken and fish. Before putting their protein on a prepared grill, novices can marinate it in tasty, low-sodium marinades. This technique not only improves the food's flavor but also keeps the vital proteins and nutrients intact.

Preserving Nutrients During Cooking:

For people on a Muscular Degeneration diet, maintaining the nutritional integrity of ingredients during cooking is crucial. Cooks who are just starting can do this by implementing certain procedures that protect the vital vitamins and minerals included in their ingredients.

First things first, it's important to use as little heat as possible and prepare food for longer periods. Vegetables in particular might lose their delicate nutrients due to overcooking. It is recommended that beginners use shorter cooking times so that the vegetables stay bright and crunchy. This can be accomplished by using rapid stir-frying or blanching methods and keeping a careful eye on the cooking process.

Furthermore, using less water when cooking can aid in the retention of nutrients. Vitamins that are soluble in water may seep into the liquid when vegetables are boiled in significant amounts of water. To counter this, novices can use just enough water to cover the vegetables or try other techniques like steaming or microwaving, which use less water and minimize the chance of losing nutrients.

Meal planning is another important aspect of preserving the integrity of vitamins and minerals. Novices should strive to eat a range of vibrant fruits and vegetables because different hues frequently indicate distinct nutrient profiles. This method contributes to the general health of the eyes by guaranteeing a wide range of vital vitamins and antioxidants.

In conclusion, beginners on a Muscular Degeneration diet must gradually learn how to use the best cooking techniques and preserve nutrients during the cooking process.

Novice cooks can produce tasty, nutrient-dense meals that support overall health and well-being by adopting methods like steaming, grilling, and sautéing with healthy oils. They can also cook mindfully by reducing heat exposure and using less water.

CHAPTER FIVE

SUPERFOODS FOR EYE HEALTH

Highlight: Foods That Help Prevent Muscular Degeneration

A frequent disorder of the eyes that affects central vision and can cause considerable vision loss is age-related macular degeneration or AMD. Thankfully, consuming a diet high in superfoods can help preserve eye health and possibly halt the advancement of AMD. Let's examine the science underlying the health advantages of some of these superfoods.

First and foremost, a major factor in supporting eye health is the consumption of leafy green vegetables like kale and spinach. Lutein and zeaxanthin, two antioxidants that build up in the retina and aid in preventing oxidative damage, are prevalent in these greens. Increasing your daily intake of leafy greens gives you a significant increase in these vital nutrients, which are especially helpful in preventing AMD.

Leafy greens are not the only foods high in omega-3 fatty acids; salmon and trout, in particular, are high in DHA and EPA. These fats are essential to the retina because they support general eye health and help maintain cell membranes. Frequent fatty fish consumption—at least two meals per week—can greatly lower the chance that AMD may advance.

Another category of superfoods that should be included in your diet to prevent muscle degeneration is nuts and seeds. Rich in zinc, important fatty acids, and vitamin E, almonds, walnuts, and flaxseeds all contribute significantly to the health of your eyes. Zinc aids in maintaining the structure of the eye, while vitamin E in particular functions as a strong antioxidant that shields cells from oxidative stress.

Strawberries and blueberries are two examples of fruits that are not only tasty but also good for your eyes. Antioxidants called anthocyanins, which are abundant in these fruits, have been connected to better night vision and a lower risk of AMD. Incorporating a range of berries into your diet not only fulfills your desire for sugar but also offers a vibrant spectrum of nutrients that are essential for preserving eye health.

Let's now focus on eggs, a superfood that is both accessible and adaptable. Like leafy greens, eggs are a good source of lutein and zeaxanthin and may be easily incorporated into a variety of meals. Eating eggs, whether poached, scrambled, or as part of a veggie omelet, is a quick and easy approach to increasing your consumption of these vital nutrients that protect your eyes.

The importance of eating a diverse range of these superfoods as part of a well-rounded diet cannot be overstated. You can be sure you're getting the full range of vitamins, minerals, and antioxidants needed to keep your eyes healthy with a varied and colorful plate. Including these foods in your regular meals might seem like a difficult endeavor at first, but you can effectively support your eye health by changing your diet with some careful preparation and inventive ideas.

How to Use Superfoods in Your Diet in a Practical Way:

Starting a diet that targets muscle atrophy can be intimidating, but with doable tactics and easy recipes, adding superfoods to your meals becomes a fun and doable task.

Leafy greens should first be incorporated into your diet gradually. Think about mixing some spinach or kale into salads or including a handful in your morning smoothie. By combining these greens with tasty foods like avocados, cherry tomatoes, and a drizzle of olive oil, you may improve the meal's nutritional content in addition to its flavor.

You can incorporate fatty fish, like salmon, into your diet with ease by using delectable recipes. For a quick and healthy supper, try baking or grilling salmon fillets seasoned with lemon and herbs. Instead, look into canned salmon options for easy lunches. You can even add them to salads or wraps for a visually appealing and filling dinner.

Nuts and seeds can be added to a wide variety of meals and snacks. Think about adding some almond or walnut crumbs to your porridge or yogurt in the morning. Throughout the day, munching on a variety of seeds—like chia and flaxseeds—offers a nutrient-rich, crunchy snack that promotes eye health.

Berries are a delightful and revitalizing method to sate your appetites and improve the health of your eyes. Enjoy a bowl of mixed berries as a dessert or snack, or blend blueberries into smoothies or yogurt. A varied intake of vitamins and antioxidants can be achieved by experimenting with different fruit combinations.

Due to their natural adaptability, eggs are a simple addition to a variety of dishes. For a quick and wholesome dinner, make a stir-fry with vegetables and eggs. For breakfast, prepare a veggie omelet. For lunch, add cooked eggs to salads. Because eggs are so versatile, you can try out several recipes until you find one that works for you.

Plan your meals to guarantee a complete and well-rounded diet. Plan a weekly menu that includes a selection of superfoods to make sure you get the full spectrum of nutrients that are essential for healthy eyes. This method not only makes grocery shopping easier but also ensures that you are getting a balanced dose of vital vitamins and minerals.

As such, implementing a diet targeted at muscle deterioration doesn't have to be difficult. It's possible to make a positive and attainable lifestyle shift by adding superfoods to your meals methodically and gradually. You may proactively support your eye health and potentially slow down the onset of age-related macular degeneration by experimenting with recipes, meal planning, and enjoying the variety these superfoods offer.

CHAPTER SIX

RECIPES FOR BREAKFAST

Easy and Packed with Nutrients Breakfast Ideas

When it comes to a Muscular Degeneration Diet, eating nutrient-dense breakfast foods first is essential to keeping your eyes as healthy as possible. Even for people with little experience in the kitchen, these simple and quick meals can be quickly included in a daily routine.

1. Berries with Overnight Oats:

Make your overnight oats with berries to start your day full of nutrition. This is an easy recipe that works well even without much effort if you make it the night before. First, in a sealed container, combine rolled oats with your preferred milk or a dairy-free substitute. Add a few handfuls of berries, like raspberries or blueberries that are high in antioxidants.

47

Overnight, the liquid is absorbed by the oats, giving them a wonderfully creamy texture in the morning. In addition to being high in fiber, this meal offers vital vitamins and minerals that promote eye health.

2. Toast with avocado and smoked salmon:

Enjoy smoked salmon on top of avocado toast for a savory take on breakfast. Omega-3 fatty acids, which are good for eye health, are among the many healthful fats found in avocados, which are a fruit high in nutrients. Just spread some ripe avocado on whole-grain toast by mashing it. Add slices of smoked salmon, which is high in protein, antioxidants, and omega-3 fatty acids. This filling breakfast option is not only delicious but also beneficial to your eyes' general health.

3. Greek Yogurt Concession:

Try this visually appealing Greek yogurt parfait to add some extra nutrition to your morning routine. Zinc, which is necessary to keep the retina healthy, is found in Greek yogurt, a food that is high in protein. To make this parfait, top Greek yogurt with fresh, vitamin C-rich fruits like kiwis, then garnish with a sprinkling of almonds or seeds for crunch. This delicious combo not only pleases your palate but also provides the nutrients your eyes need to function at their best.

4. Mixed Fruit Chia Seed Pudding:

Enjoy a chia seed pudding full of mixed fruit delights to invigorate your mornings. Chia seeds support heart and eye health since they are high in fiber and omega-3 fatty acids. This nutrient-dense pudding may be made by combining chia seeds with your preferred milk and refrigerating it overnight. Place a mixture of mixed fruits, such as mango, pomegranate seeds, and kiwis, on top of the pudding in the morning. This breakfast alternative gives your eyes a burst of vital nutrients while also satisfying your sweet needs.

5. Breakfast Bowl with Quinoa:

A quinoa bowl that mixes protein-rich quinoa with a range of visually appealing toppings will up your morning game. Prepare the quinoa as directed on the package, then garnish with chopped nuts, such as almonds or walnuts, sliced bananas, and honey. Vitamin A, which is essential for preserving good vision, is abundant in bananas. Quinoa and almonds work together to give a delightful crunch and provide vital nutrients that promote the health of your eyes.

6. Breakfast hash with sweet potatoes and spinach:

Add some nutrients to your morning routine by making a breakfast hash made of sweet potatoes and spinach. Beta-carotene, which is a precursor to vitamin A, is abundant in sweet potatoes, and lutein and zeaxanthin, which are vital for eye health, are found in spinach.

Diced sweet potatoes should be sautéed in olive oil until golden brown before serving this hearty breakfast. Cook the fresh spinach until it wilts. For more taste, season with your preferred herbs and spices. In addition to being delicious, this substantial and nutrient-rich morning hash improves the general health of your eyes.

Including these simple, high-nutrient breakfast choices in your Muscular Degeneration Diet guarantees a healthy start to your day, which promotes long-term energy and improved eye health.

Smoothies for Breakfast to Promote Eye Health

Smoothies are a delicious way to start the day and help you stick to your muscle degeneration diet. These breakfast smoothies are not only simple to make but also full of vital nutrients that help support eye health.

1. Smoothie with Berry Blast:

Blend a handful of mixed berries, including strawberries, blueberries, and blackberries, to make a colorful and antioxidant-rich smoothie. These berries are packed with vitamins, including C and anthocyanins, which are linked to eye protection. To make a dairy-free base, add a splash of almond milk, a scoop of Greek yogurt for protein, and a banana for richness. You'll have a tasty morning smoothie that promotes the health of your eyes after blending until smooth.

2. Healthy Green Smoothie:

Put leafy greens to use by making a Green Bliss smoothie. Rich in lutein and zeaxanthin, two important antioxidants that support eye health, are kale and spinach. A ripe banana, a piece of pineapple for sweetness, and coconut water for hydration should all be combined with a handful of these greens. Blend until you have a smooth consistency. This nutrient-dense smoothie provides vital vitamins and minerals to support your eyes in addition to satisfying your taste senses.

3. Smoothie with Tropical Delight:

Smoothie that blends the goodness of tropical fruits and takes your taste senses to a tropical paradise. Mango, pineapple, and papaya can be blended to create a tasty base that is high in vitamins A and C. For fiber and omega-3 fatty acids, add a scoop of chia seeds. Add a handful of goji berries, which are well-known for having a high antioxidant content, to increase the benefits to eye health. In addition to providing a taste explosion of exotic flavors, this tropical delight smoothie helps you achieve your Muscular Degeneration Diet objectives.

4. Orange Flavor Smoothie:

Make a delicious citrus smoothie to start your day with a burst of lemony goodness. Vitamin C, a potent antioxidant that promotes the health of your eyes, may be found in abundance in oranges, grapefruits, and tangerines. Add some spinach for extra nutrients, a banana for creaminess, and coconut water for hydration to this citrus fruit and banana combo. Blend until smooth. You'll have a vibrant, nutrient-rich smoothie that will excite your taste buds and supply vital vitamins for the best possible eye health.

5. Smoothie with almond butter and banana bliss:

Savor a smooth and fulfilling smoothie made with almond butter and bananas that blends the healthy potassium content of bananas with the rich flavor of almond butter. Almond butter is an excellent source of healthy fats and vitamin E, which help to maintain eye health. Blend a ripe banana, a dollop of almond butter, a little almond milk, and Greek yogurt for extra protein. The outcome is a rich, nutrient-rich smoothie that not only quells your hunger but also provides your eyes with much-needed nourishment.

6. Berry Smoothie with Antioxidant Powerhouse:

Upgrade your morning routine with a berry smoothie that is a powerhouse of antioxidants and incorporates a range of berries that have been linked to eye protection. For an added antioxidant boost, blend blackberries, blueberries, and strawberries with a scoop of acai berry puree. Add some almond milk for a smooth consistency, some kale for extra nutrients, and a banana for sweetness. In addition to satisfying your appetite, this colorful and delectable smoothie provides a strong antioxidant boost to help your Muscular Degeneration Diet.

If you include these smoothies for breakfast every day, you'll have a tasty and easy method to get the vital nutrients your eyes need to stay healthy and your Muscular Degeneration Diet fun.

CHAPTER SEVEN

SNACKS AT LUNCH

Simple Lunch Recipes to Make:

Prioritizing simplicity and nutritional value is a good idea when developing lunch foods that are simple to make and fit into a muscle degeneration diet. These recipes are designed to make eating enjoyable while guaranteeing that the ingredients are not only tasty but also have a beneficial effect on eye health.

Quinoa with a Veggie Salad:

First up, here's a simple but filling dish: quinoa and vegetable salad. This recipe mixes a colorful assortment of veggies with the health benefits of quinoa, a grain high in protein. To start, give the quinoa a thorough rinse to get rid of any bitterness. Cook it as directed on the package, then let it cool. Combine the cooked quinoa, cucumber, spinach, cherry tomatoes, and finely diced bell peppers in a big bowl. The vivid hues of the meal not only enhance its visual appeal but also represent a variety of nutrients. Use a simple vinaigrette composed of lemon juice, olive oil, and a small amount of herbs to dress the salad. This light salad offers a balanced combination of important nutrients and protective antioxidants to maintain eye health.

Vegetable And Lentil Stew:

For a warm alternative, think about making a vegetable and lentil stew. This robust stew has a high protein and fiber content and is rather simple to prepare. In a pot, start by sautéing the onions and garlic until aromatic. Add the chopped zucchini, celery, and carrots, and let them soften. Before adding green or brown lentils to the saucepan, rinse and drain them. Add a blend of herbs, such as thyme and rosemary, to the vegetable broth to enhance its flavor. Once the vegetables are perfectly cooked and the lentils are soft, simmer the stew. This hearty and nourishing stew can become a lunchtime mainstay, enhancing eye health and fostering general well-being.

Buddha Bowl with Sweet Potato and Chickpeas:

Sweet potatoes, chickpeas, and a rainbow of colorful vegetables come together to create this brilliant Buddha Bowl. To enhance the taste, begin by roasting sweet potatoes in diced form, sprinkling with smoked paprika and a splash of olive oil. In the meantime, roast a batch of chickpeas until they get crispy by tossing them in a mixture of cumin, coriander, and a little olive oil. Put the roasted sweet potatoes and chickpeas in a bowl and top with shredded kale, avocado slices, and fresh cherry tomatoes. Finish with a creamy and nutrient-dense dressing made with tahini. In addition to being bursting with flavor, this Buddha Bowl provides an abundance of vitamins and antioxidants that are critical for eye health.

Quinoa-stuffed peppers with salmon:

Enjoy a more satisfying lunch with salmon and quinoa stuffed peppers, a high-protein and omega-3 fatty acid meal. Cook the quinoa per the directions on the package to start. Diced onions, garlic, and spinach should be sautéed until wilted in a separate pan. Stir the cooked quinoa into the sautéed vegetable mixture, flake salmon, and lemon zest for color. Bell peppers make ideal receptacles for the stuffing when they are cut in half and the seeds removed. After filling the pepper halves with the quinoa and salmon mixture, roast the peppers until they are soft. In addition to pleasing your palate, this vibrant and tasty dish offers vital nutrients that support eye health.

Mediterranean Salad with Chickpeas:

Enjoy the tastes of the Mediterranean with this nutrient-dense, cool chickpea salad. Rinse and drain the canned chickpeas first. Combine the chickpeas, cucumber, red onion, cherry tomatoes, and Kalamata olives in a big bowl. Add chopped fresh parsley and crumbled feta cheese to intensify the taste. Mix extra virgin olive oil, lemon juice, minced garlic, and a dash of oregano to make a dressing and drizzle it over the salad. To guarantee an even coating, combine everything. In addition to offering a plethora of tastes, this Mediterranean Chickpea Salad is packed with antioxidants, vitamins, and minerals that support eye health.

These extra Simple Lunch Recipes are packed with nutrients and a variety of flavors, which makes them perfect for anyone on a diet that prevents muscle atrophy. These recipes promote eye health and general well-being in a tasty and approachable way by using nutrient-dense foods, lean meats, and colorful veggies.

Including Lean Proteins and Vibrant Vegetables:

When searching for dishes that address muscle atrophy, including colorful veggies and lean meats becomes essential. These ingredients improve the appearance of your food while also adding to a diet that is nutrient-dense and well-balanced, which is necessary to preserve good eye health.

Let's explore the world of vibrant veggies and how to include them in your meals smoothly and easily. To make a Rainbow Veggie Stir-Fry is a quick and easy way. Begin by choosing a variety of colorful veggies, including bell peppers, broccoli, carrots, and snap peas. To guarantee even cooking, chop them into uniform-sized pieces. Ginger and garlic should be sautéed in a little olive oil in a hot pan. Stir-fry the vegetables until they become bright and slightly crisp, starting with the ones that require longer to cook. Add a sauce consisting of low-sodium soy sauce, ginger, and a small amount of honey to bring out the flavors. In addition to being visually appealing, this quick and colorful stir-fry offers a variety of nutrients that are good for eye health.

Let's now discuss the inclusion of lean proteins, which is an essential component of the diet for muscle deterioration. A delicious choice that combines the health benefits of lean protein with the zesty freshness of herbs is grilled lemon herb chicken breast. Start by marinating chicken breasts in a concoction of olive oil, lemon juice, minced garlic, and a mixture of herbs, including thyme and rosemary. To fully infuse the flavors, let the chicken marinate for at least thirty minutes. Before cooking the chicken breasts, preheat the grill and cook them until the inside is cooked through and the outside is golden brown. In addition to pleasing the palate, this dish's flavorful simplicity provides vital nutrients that promote eye health.

For beginners who want to follow a muscular degeneration diet, these simple lunch recipes along with the addition of colorful veggies and lean proteins offer a useful and guided approach. A fulfilling and visually appealing culinary adventure can be paved with these recipes' emphasis on simplicity, colorful ingredients, and balanced nutrition.

CHAPTER EIGHT

HEALTHFUL DINNERS FOR OPTICAL HEALTH
Recipes for Dinner That Highlight Nutrient-Rich Ingredients

Starting on a path to maintain eye health with a diet designed for macular degeneration entails adding foods high in nutrients to your dinners. Not only are these ingredients tasty, but they are also a great source of vital vitamins and minerals that support eye health.

Begin with a base of leafy greens, high in lutein and zeaxanthin, like kale and spinach. These antioxidants can help preserve good vision and have been connected to a decreased risk of macular degeneration. Making a colorful salad with veggies like tomatoes, carrots, and bell peppers is an easy way to incorporate these greens. Add a small amount of nuts, like walnuts or almonds, to get your fill of omega-3 fatty acids, which are good for your eyes.

Include lean proteins in your meals, such as trout or salmon, as they are great providers of astaxanthin and omega-3 fatty acids, which may help shield the eyes from oxidative damage. A simple and delectable way to prepare these fish is to grill or bake them. Furthermore, take into account adding brown rice or quinoa as a healthy source of fiber that can improve general health and possibly lower the risk of age-related macular degeneration.

Try experimenting with herbs and spices like turmeric, which has anti-inflammatory qualities, to add taste and extra health benefits. For a tasty and nutritious supper, make a stir-fried stir-fried chicken or vegetables with turmeric. Curcumin, the active ingredient in turmeric, has demonstrated the potential to enhance eye health by lowering oxidative stress and inflammation.

One-Pot Dinners for Ease

One-pot meals are a practical and effective choice for people who are juggling a busy schedule or are just beginning their culinary adventure.

These recipes make cooking easier and require less cleanup, which makes them perfect for novice and seasoned cooks alike.

One-pot options that are filling and hearty are lentil and vegetable stews. Lentils are full of nutrient-dense vegetables and are a great source of fiber, protein, and important vitamins. Before adding lentils and broth, this stew can be quickly made by sautéing onions, garlic, and a variety of colorful vegetables. Give the ingredients a little time to simmer, and you'll have a nutritious, visually appealing dinner in no time.

A favorite one-pot meal is a skillet of vegetables and quinoa. Start by sautéing a variety of vegetables, such as cherry tomatoes, bell peppers, and zucchini. When the quinoa is cooked and has absorbed the flavors, add the rinsed quinoa and vegetable broth to the skillet and let it simmer. This tasty and easy recipe offers a good balance of antioxidants, fiber, and protein.

For dinner, consider a quick sheet pan meal of salmon or trout with a rainbow of colorful vegetables. Arrange vegetables on a baking sheet around the fish, tossing them in olive oil and seasonings. This includes asparagus, sweet potatoes, and cherry tomatoes. All of the ingredients can be roasted together to create a simple, yet nutrient-dense meal that promotes eye health because it contains omega-3 fatty acids and several vitamins.

More Dinner Recipes Packed with Nutrients:

1. Chicken Breast Stuffed with Spinach and Mushrooms:

The lean protein of chicken breast is combined with the health benefits of spinach and mushrooms in this tasty and nutrient-rich dish. First, release the moisture and soften the spinach and mushrooms by sautéing them in olive oil with finely chopped mushrooms. Using a butterfly, make a pocket in the chicken breasts for stuffing. Sprinkle some salt, pepper, and garlic powder inside the chicken. Place toothpicks inside each breast after stuffing it with the sautéed mushroom and spinach mixture. Bake the chicken for the entire cooking time in the oven. In addition to being a filling meal, this dish provides important vitamins and minerals that support eye health.

2. Bell peppers stuffed with quinoa and kale:

These quinoa and kale stuffed bell peppers are a nutrient-dense, high-fiber, antioxidant, and vitamin-rich option that will elevate your dinner. Follow the directions on the package to cook the quinoa. Add the diced tomatoes, chopped kale, and black beans to a pan and cook until the kale wilts. Stir in the cooked quinoa and the sautéed mixture; add salt, chili powder, and cumin for seasoning. Halve the bell peppers and remove the seeds to make a hollow that can hold the stuffing. After filling the pepper halves with the quinoa and kale mixture, bake the peppers until they are soft. This vibrant and filling dish promotes general health and healthy eye function in addition to satisfying your appetite.

3. Salmon baked in a pan with roasted veggies:

Baked salmon and a medley of roasted vegetables make for a tasty and nutrient-dense supper. To begin, rub salmon fillets with a mixture of dill, garlic, olive oil, and lemon juice. Arrange the salmon onto a parchment paper-lined baking sheet. Toss a variety of colorful veggies, like bell peppers, cherry tomatoes, and asparagus, with olive oil, salt, and pepper in a separate bowl. On the baking sheet, arrange the vegetables around the salmon. Bake until the vegetables are perfectly roasted and the salmon is flaky. This dinner option offers a variety of vitamins and minerals that are good for keeping the eye healthy in addition to a substantial dose of omega-3 fatty acids.

These tasty and useful dinner recipes are a great way to add important vitamins, minerals, and antioxidants to your diet. These recipes, which emphasize lean proteins, whole grains, and vibrant vegetables, enhance general health and cater to the dietary requirements of those who follow a muscular degeneration diet.

You can incorporate visually appealing dinners into your routine with ease if you prioritize using nutrient-dense ingredients and embrace the ease of preparation of one-pot meals. These recipes not only improve your general health but also make cooking fun for beginners, making for a fulfilling and health-conscious mealtime experience.

CHAPTER NINE

EFFICIENT SNACKING

Snack Ideas That Are Healthier and Promote Eye Health

Eating a diet that promotes muscle preservation requires making a deliberate effort to include snacks that are especially beneficial to eye health. These snacks fulfill your cravings while also giving your eyes the vital nutrients they need to stay healthy. Here's how to add nutritious snack options to your daily routine step-by-step:

1. **Accept Nutrient-rich fruits and Vegetables:** Begin by including a range of fruits and vegetables that are high in antioxidants, vitamins, and minerals. Vegetables like bell peppers, sweet potatoes, carrots, and spinach are great options. These foods include important nutrients that are known to support eye health, like lutein, beta-carotene, and vitamin C.

2. Examine Nuts and Seeds: Rich in vitamin E and omega-3 fatty acids, which support eye health, nuts and seeds are nutrient-dense power snacks. Nuts like flaxseeds, chia seeds, walnuts, and almonds are excellent choices. For a quick and nutrient-dense snack, try mixing these nuts and seeds into a trail mix.

3. Include Whole Grains: For a consistent energy release and long-lasting satiety, opt for whole grains rather than refined ones. Nutrients like zinc and niacin found in whole grains like quinoa, brown rice, and oats promote general eye health. For a filling snack, try whole-grain crackers or rice cakes with a healthy topping like avocado or hummus.

4. Incorporate Lean Proteins: The health of your muscles, including the muscles in your eyes, depends on getting enough lean protein. Add in some snacks, such as hard-boiled eggs, lean turkey slices, or Greek yogurt. These offer essential nutrients like zinc and selenium in addition to protein, which helps to maintain the best possible eye function.

5. Expand Your Diet by Including Dairy or Dairy Alternatives: Calcium and vitamin D are essential for good health in general, which includes healthy eyes. Think about expanding your snack options to include fortified dairy substitutes or low-fat dairy products. Smoothies made with enhanced almond milk or Greek yogurt topped with fresh berries can be incredibly tasty and nourishing.

6. Drink Herbal Teas and Infusions to Stay Hydrated: Maintaining proper hydration is crucial for eye health. Herbal infusions and teas offer antioxidants that support eye health in addition to being hydrating. Green tea, chamomile tea, or a cool concoction of cucumber and mint can be tasty options for sensible snacking.

7. Mindful Portion Control: To prevent overindulging, be mindful of portion sizes. Control can be preserved by preparing snacks in tiny, portioned containers. This keeps you from consuming extra calories and guarantees that you get the proper ratio of nutrients for good eye health.

You're not only pleasing your palate by including these nutrient-dense snacks in your regular diet, but you're also giving your eyes the vital nutrients they require to remain healthy.

Steer clear of processed snacks and sweet treats

Avoiding processed foods and sweets is a key component of a diet that prevents muscle atrophy. Processed snacks can cause inflammation and have a detrimental effect on eye health because they frequently include unhealthy fats, too much salt, and artificial additives. Here's a step-by-step guide to help you cut these unhealthy snacks from your diet and make wise decisions:

1. **Read Food Labels Mindfully:** Make it a habit to carefully read food labels. Keep an eye out for substances like high-fructose corn syrup, trans fats, and excess sodium. Choose whole foods or

minimally processed snacks to make sure you're not inadvertently consuming unhealthy additives.

2. Select Whole, Unprocessed Foods: Giving priority to whole, unprocessed foods is a crucial first step in steering clear of processed snacks. Your best bet should be fresh fruits, vegetables, nuts, and seeds. Without the added sugars and unhealthy fats present in many processed snacks, these foods offer vital nutrients.

3. Make Your Snack Alternatives: Become in charge of the snacks you eat by making your alternatives. Make your trail mix by combining dried fruits, seeds, and raw nuts. You can control the ingredients when you bake kale chips or whole-grain crackers at home, guaranteeing a healthy and nutrient-dense snack.

4. Choose Natural, Fresh Sweeteners: If you're craving something sweet, go for naturally sweet options. A drizzle of honey, fresh fruits, or dried fruits free of added sugars can be healthier substitutes for processed sweets. These options offer antioxidants and vitamins that are good for the health of the eyes along with sweetness.

5. Conscientious Substitutions: When you're in the mood for something salty, choose snacks that have a nice crunch without being overly high in fat or sodium. Use baked sweet potato or kale chips in place of regular chips. With this easy replacement, you can increase the nutritional content of your snacks without sacrificing crunch.

6. Limit Sugary Beverages: Sugary beverages and processed snacks frequently go hand in hand, leading to excessive calorie intake and possible health problems. Instead of sugary drinks, opt for infused water, herbal teas, or water. Using these choices to stay hydrated promotes general health, which includes eye health.

7. Moderation is key, even though it's important to stay away from processed snacks and sugary treats. Abruptly cutting yourself off could result in cravings and possibly binge eating. Treats are fine once in a while, just make sure they're balanced and part of your overall healthy diet.

You can gradually cut out processed snacks and sugary treats from your diet by intentionally making these decisions.

Emphasizing complete, nutrient-dense foods will benefit your general health in addition to eye health.

CHAPTER TEN

DESSERTS WITH A PURPOSE

Sweets that Complement a Dietary Approach to Muscular Degeneration:

Sweet treats don't always have to be a guilty pleasure, especially if you're on a diet that prevents muscular degeneration. This particular diet places a strong emphasis on nutrient-dense foods that promote general health and eye health. It may seem difficult to include sweets in this diet, but you can have desserts that fit your needs if you choose the right ingredients and make thoughtful decisions.

Start by choosing fruits high in antioxidants, like berries, which have been demonstrated to promote eye health. Try assembling a colorful fruit salad with blueberries, strawberries, and kiwis, among other vibrant fruits.

These fruits provide necessary vitamins and minerals in addition to satisfying your sweet tooth.

Yogurt parfait with a twist is another delicious option. Arrange fresh fruits and granola on top of a low-fat plain yogurt. Yogurt supplies calcium and the granola gives it a delightful crunch. This dessert offers a delicious blend of flavors and textures in addition to being in line with the Muscular Degeneration Diet.

Experimenting with healthy dessert smoothies can also be a rewarding venture. Blend frozen fruits like mangoes, pineapples, and bananas with a base of almond milk or Greek yogurt. The result is a creamy, delicious smoothie packed with vitamins and antioxidants. Adding a handful of spinach can further enhance the nutritional value without compromising the flavor.

For those with a sweet tooth, consider baking oatmeal cookies with a Muscular Degeneration Diet-friendly twist. Use whole-grain oats, and mashed bananas as a natural sweetener, and incorporate chopped nuts for added crunch and nutrients. This alternative ensures that you enjoy a satisfying dessert without compromising on your dietary goals.

Dessert Substitutes for Healthier Options:

Finding healthier alternatives to typical desserts is an important element of the Muscular Degeneration Diet. One feasible solution is to replace processed sugars with natural sweeteners like honey or maple syrup. These alternatives not only add sweetness to your desserts but also provide additional minerals and antioxidants.

When it comes to baking, consider utilizing whole-grain flour instead of refined white flour. Whole-grain flours, such as whole wheat or almond flour, offer a nutty flavor and improve the fiber content of your desserts. Experimenting with different flours may require some tweaking, but the result is a healthy treat that corresponds with the Muscular Degeneration Diet.

Explore the world of plant-based desserts as another replacement choice. Avocado-based chocolate mousse or coconut milk-based ice cream can be excellent alternatives that are rich in healthy fats and devoid of dairy. These solutions not only cater to people following a vegan diet but also provide a creamy and pleasing feel.

Swap your typical high-fat items with healthy alternatives in your dessert recipes. For example, use Greek yogurt instead of heavy cream or butter to produce creamy sweets. This easy adjustment minimizes saturated fat intake while adding protein to your sweet sweets.

Incorporating nuts and seeds into your sweets is another smart idea. These components not only contribute to texture but also bring a plethora of health advantages. Almonds, walnuts, and chia seeds, for instance, supply good fats and omega-3 fatty acids, promoting general eye health in alignment with the Muscular Degeneration Diet.

Therefore, with a thorough approach to item selection and preparation procedures, you can enjoy sweet pleasures that not only satisfy your needs but also correspond with the Muscular

Degeneration Diet. By adopting these dessert replacements and healthier options, you can make tasty choices that contribute to your overall well-being while indulging in the enjoyment of a sweet treat.

CHAPTER ELEVEN

DINING OUT AND SOCIAL SITUATIONS
Navigating Restaurants with a Muscular Degeneration Diet

Navigating restaurants with a muscle degeneration diet can be a tough but manageable process with proper planning and informed decisions. Whether you're a rookie or someone accustomed to dietary restrictions due to muscle degeneration, it's vital to approach dining out with a strategic perspective. This requires recognizing your nutritional requirements, communicating them effectively, and making informed decisions that match your health goals.

To begin with, it's vital to investigate and select eateries that offer a variety of selections ideal for a muscle degeneration diet. Many restaurants now give nutritional information on their menus or websites, making it easier for individuals with specific dietary needs to make informed judgments. Utilizing internet tools or calling ahead to check about menu alternatives might be a beneficial first step. Look for restaurants that stress fresh, nutrient-rich products and are willing to accommodate particular dietary demands.

When you arrive at the restaurant, take your time examining the menu. Focus on foods that highlight lean proteins, vegetables, and nutritious grains. Steer wary of things that are deep-fried, too high in saturated fats, or laden with sodium. Many restaurants are happy to alter meals to fit dietary restrictions, so don't hesitate to ask for tweaks or substitutions to better align with your muscle degeneration diet.

Communication is crucial when dining out with certain dietary demands. When ordering, properly state your requirements to the server, highlighting any restrictions or preferences. For example, if you need your meal made with little added salt or certain cooking methods, don't hesitate to communicate this information to the kitchen staff.

Being proactive and outspoken about your dietary preferences will assist create a more pleasurable dining experience.

Additionally, consider choosing appetizers or sides as these generally offer more versatility for customizing. By creating a meal from these components, you can make a dish that meets your muscle degeneration diet without feeling confined. It's crucial to stay open-minded and be willing to explore numerous menu selections to find combinations that both delight your taste buds and conform to your dietary limitations.

Making Informed Choices at Social Gatherings

When attending social gatherings, such as parties or events, it's useful to plan. If possible, inquire about the food beforehand and explain your dietary demands to the host or caterer. This proactive strategy can considerably boost the likelihood of having adequate meal alternatives accessible, decreasing any potential stress or pain during the occasion.

At social occasions, focus on constructing a well-balanced dish with a combination of lean proteins, colorful veggies, and complete grains. Avoid excessively processed or fried foods, and be aware of portion amounts. If you're confused about the ingredients in a particular meal, don't hesitate to contact the host or catering staff for further information. Most people are accommodating and sympathetic when it comes to dietary restrictions, and taking the initiative to convey your needs can lead to a more enjoyable experience for everyone involved.

Therefore, navigating restaurants and social situations with a muscle degeneration diet takes careful planning, informed decision-making, and good communication. By researching menus, making strategic selections, and explaining your dietary preferences, you can enjoy dining out and socializing while adhering to your health goals. Approach each circumstance with confidence, and don't be hesitant to fight for your dietary preferences to create a great and satisfying experience.

CHAPTER TWELVE

NUTRITIONAL SUPPLEMENTS AND THEIR ROLE

Comprehending Supplementary Choices:

When entering into the domain of nutritional supplements for a Muscular Degeneration Diet Cookbook, it's vital to comprehend the plethora of possibilities available. Supplements can play a crucial role in maintaining eye health and general well-being. The trick lies in understanding what each supplement brings to the table and how it complements the nutritional needs associated with muscle degeneration.

First and foremost, consider including antioxidants in the program. These strong substances, such as vitamins A, C, and E, as well as zinc and copper, help battle oxidative stress that contributes to muscle degeneration.

Selecting a high-quality multivitamin specialized for eye health helps ease the process, guaranteeing a full intake of these critical antioxidants.

Omega-3 fatty acids, notably docosahexaenoic acid (DHA) and eicosapentaenoic acid (EPA) demand special attention. Found abundantly in fish oil supplements, these fatty acids are recognized for their anti-inflammatory characteristics, which can be effective in regulating and preventing muscle deterioration. Consider fish oil capsules or explore plant-based options like algal oil for individuals who want a vegetarian or vegan approach.

Lutein and zeaxanthin, carotenoids present in high concentrations in the retina, are necessary for sustaining good eyesight. These molecules operate as natural filters, protecting the eyes from damaging high-energy light waves like UV radiation. Selecting supplements rich in lutein and zeaxanthin, or researching sources like marigold flower extract, can boost their presence in the diet.

Another helpful addition to the supplement repertoire is Coenzyme Q10 (CoQ10). This enzyme, naturally produced by the body, declines with age, influencing cellular energy generation. Supplementing with CoQ10 can support mitochondrial function, potentially slowing down degenerative processes.

Vitamin B complex is also of significance. B vitamins—B6, B9 (folate), and B12—help maintain healthy eyes and lower homocysteine levels, which are linked to a higher risk of muscle degeneration. It is crucial to make sure that you are getting enough of these B vitamins from your food or supplements.

It's important to be aware of potential interactions and contraindications when navigating the world of supplements. It's critical to know the recommended dosage for each supplement and to take any current medical conditions or prescription drugs into account. Always choose trustworthy, high-quality products to guarantee potency and purity.

Seeking Advice from a Medical Professional:

Deciding to include dietary supplements in a Muscular Degeneration Diet Cookbook is something that should be carefully thought through and, most importantly, discussed with a healthcare provider. This is not simply a formality; it's an important part of making sure the supplements meet specific health demands and don't conflict with prescription drugs or pre-existing medical issues.

Make an extensive consultation with an eye care specialist or general healthcare physician before beginning any supplementation routine. Be transparent while discussing the plan to add supplements to the diet and the particular issues surrounding the deterioration of the muscles. By taking this proactive measure, the medical practitioner can customize advice according to the patient's health profile.

Give a thorough medical history during the consultation, mentioning any current eye diseases, prescription drugs, food allergies, or dietary restrictions. The healthcare provider can provide tailored suggestions with this thorough assessment, guaranteeing that the supplements chosen meet individual needs and complement the entire health plan.

Ask questions regarding possible interactions, side effects, and the best dosage for each supplement when you're talking about them. A healthcare practitioner can help people make educated decisions by guiding them away from misinformation and providing insights into the most recent study findings.

In other instances, medical professionals could suggest specific eye examinations or tests to determine the degree of muscle deterioration and adjust the supplement regimen accordingly. This focused method guarantees that the selected supplements meet the unique needs of the person, enhancing their effectiveness.

Furthermore, to track the results and modify the supplement regimen as needed, follow-up sessions at regular intervals are essential. Medical practitioners can monitor changes in ocular health, handle new issues, and adjust the strategy for the best outcomes.

Consequently, seeking advice from a medical expert is not only a wise precaution but also a crucial component of creating a comprehensive and successful Muscular Degeneration Diet Cookbook. This cooperative endeavor guarantees that the selected supplements align with personal health requirements, promoting self-assurance in the quest for ideal eye health and general well-being.

CHAPTER THIRTEEN

MAINTAINING A LIFETIME DIET FOR MUSCULAR DEGENERATION

Long-Term Dedication to Ocular Health:

Long-term adherence to a muscle degeneration diet is crucial for the general health of your eyes, not only as a short-term fix. Understanding that consistency is essential is essential to starting this journey successfully. For long-term eye health, you must establish a program that easily incorporates the required foods and exercises into your daily existence.

Learning about the precise food requirements that promote eye health is one of the first stages. You should make a range of nutrient-dense foods, like leafy greens, vibrant fruits, and omega-3 fatty acids, mainstays in your diet. Being aware of how each vitamin supports ocular function gives you the power to organize your meals with knowledge.

Consider making a weekly meal plan to make this commitment easier to maintain. By taking the initiative, you can stay organized and make sure you have all the necessary supplies on hand. Divide the schedule into four meals: breakfast, lunch, supper, and snacks. At each meal, provide a variety of nutrients. To avoid forgetting important products and to make your grocery shopping excursions easier, create a shopping list based on your meal plan.

Your long-term commitment should include frequent eye exams in addition to nutrition. Plan yearly examinations with an ophthalmologist to keep an eye on the condition of your eyes and to quickly address any new issues that may arise. Regular check-ups help to sustain your muscle degeneration diet by acting as preventive measures and enabling early intervention if needed.

Establishing a nurturing atmosphere is equally important. Encourage friends and family to join you on this journey by sharing your pledge with them.

A network of support can be very helpful in keeping you motivated and fostering a sense of community as you strive to maintain long-term excellent eye health.

Honoring Achievers and Overcoming Obstacles:

Maintaining a muscle degeneration diet requires acknowledging and appreciating accomplishments of all sizes. Acknowledging and praising yourself for sticking to your diet objectives produces positive reinforcement, increasing the likelihood that you'll stick with it in the long run.

Set attainable goals for yourself as you start this adventure. These achievements could be anything from effectively avoiding harmful temptations to regularly including particular nutrient-rich foods in your diet. Celebrate and acknowledge these successes, and continue to reinforce the good habits that support the health of your eyes.

It's crucial to recognize that difficulties could occur. Having measures in place is essential for dealing with cravings for less-than-ideal food choices and social situations where dietary restrictions may cause challenges. To keep your attention on your long-term objectives, practice mindful eating and prepare yourself with healthier alternatives for when cravings arise.

Talk to friends and family about your nutritional demands to overcome social obstacles. Tell them about the significance of your diet for preventing muscle deterioration and ask for their cooperation. Furthermore, take the initiative to seek out eateries or menu items that meet your dietary needs so that social events become chances to demonstrate your dedication to eye health rather than a barrier.

When anything goes wrong, see it as a teaching opportunity rather than a failure. Examine the reasons for the diet lapse and devise plans to deal with them moving forward. This methodical technique improves your ability to adapt to changing circumstances and fortifies your resilience.

By acknowledging your accomplishments and overcoming obstacles, you develop a positive outlook that is essential to maintaining a muscle degeneration diet over the long term. Recall that keeping your best eye health over the long run depends on you choosing to have a resilient and joyful mindset. This is a marathon, not a sprint.

MY GRATITUDES

Dear Valued Readers and Supporters,

I hope this message finds you well. I am writing to express my deepest gratitude to both God and each one of you for the overwhelming support and positive response to my book. Your encouragement and enthusiasm have truly touched my heart, and I am immensely thankful for the journey we are on together.

I believe that every success is a result of collaboration and support from various sources. First and foremost, I want to acknowledge the divine guidance and inspiration that led me to create this cookbook. Without the grace of God, this endeavor would not have been possible.

To my cherished readers, your commitment to exploring healthier dietary options for managing your crises has been both inspiring and humbling. Your trust in this book" means the world to me, and I am honored to be part of your journey toward improved health and well-being.

Also, I am reaching out to kindly request your valuable feedback on this book. Your thoughts and insights are crucial in helping me enhance and serve you better, ensuring that it continues to meet your needs effectively. Please take a moment to share your thoughts by rating and writing reviews on platforms where the book is available.

Your reviews not only provide me with invaluable feedback but also play a significant role in assisting others in making informed choices. By sharing your experiences, you contribute to a community that values health and wellness, creating a positive impact on countless lives.

Additionally, I encourage you to share this book with your friends, family and loved ones. Together, we can extend the reach of this promising resource, offering support and guidance to those who may benefit from it. Having this knowledge and seeking medical advice from your specialist I anticipate a turnaround for us.

Once again, thank you from the depths of my heart for your unwavering support. I am committed to continually improving and serving you better. Let us continue this journey together, promoting health, well-being, and a shared sense of community.

With sincere appreciation,

[Emmy Brooks]

Author, "MUSCULAR DEGENERATION DIET COOKBOOK"

www.ingramcontent.com/pod-product-compliance
Lightning Source LLC
Chambersburg PA
CBHW070748290526
45795CB00002B/528